Vegan Gluten

Nutritious and Delicious, 100% Vegan Gluten-Free Recipes to Improve Your Health, Lose Weight, and Feel Amazing

By Kira Novac (ISBN-10: 1518619606)

Copyright ©Kira Novac 2015

www.amazon.com/author/kira-novac

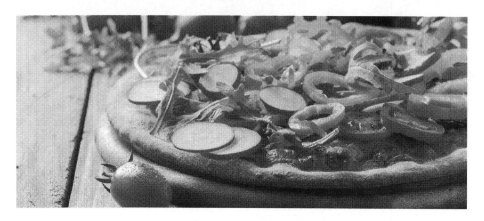

Table of contents

Introduction

When you switch to the vegan diet, you may be worried about whether or not you will still be able to eat your favorite foods. While you might have to make some big changes to your diet, there are plenty of vegan alternatives out there for traditional foods. You can still enjoy things like pancakes, muffins, even omelets for breakfast as well as hearty soups, stews, and entrees – even decadent desserts! The vegan diet is an excellent choice if you are looking for a way to improve your health and vitality and, with the recipes included in this book, you won't feel like you are making a sacrifice.

Another diet that has recently skyrocketed in popularity is the gluten-free diet. While many people are forced to switch to this diet out of medical necessity resulting from gluten allergies or intolerance, some people are making the switch simply because they think it is a healthy alternative to the modern Western diet. The truth of the matter is that the gluten-free diet is not a magical solution for weight loss or health problems, but you can use it as a tool to achieve your health and wellness goals. The gluten-free diet can even be combined with the vegan diet, if you like!

The vegan gluten-free diet might take a little bit of getting used to because you can no longer eat animal products like meat, eggs, and dairy – you also need to avoid gluten-containing grains like wheat, barley and rye. If you take the time to really learn about this diet, however, you will find that there are still plenty of vegan gluten-free options out there. You can still enjoy tasty muffins and pancakes made with gluten-free flours as well as vegan versions of your favorite soups and stews. The vegan gluten-free diet can be adapted to include everything from pasta and rice dishes to indulgent desserts.

Once you make the switch to the vegan gluten-free diet you shouldn't be surprised if you feel your body start to change. Removing processed grains and animal products from your diet can work wonders for your digestion and your body as a whole. You may find that you have more energy during the day and that you no longer suffer from food cravings. The vegan gluten-free diet can be used as a tool for weight loss because many of the foods included in the diet are naturally low in calories but high in nutrition. Just be sure to mind your portions and make an effort to follow a balanced diet.

If you are ready to give the vegan gluten-free diet a try, this book is the perfect place to start. In the pages of this book you will find a collection of dozens of vegan gluten-free recipes from oriental to traditional and everything in between.

About the Recipes

The cup measurement I use is the American cup measurement.

If you don't have American Cup measures, just use a metric or imperial liquid measuring jug and fill your jug with your ingredient to the corresponding level. Here's how to go about it:

1 American Cup = 250ml = 8 fl.oz

For example:

If a recipe calls for 1 cup of almonds, simply place your almonds into your measuring jug until it reaches the 250 ml/8oz mark.

I know that different countries use different measurements and I wanted to make things simple for you. I have also noticed that very often those who are used to American cup measurements complain about metric measurements and vice versa. However, if you apply what I have just explained, you will find it easy to use both.

Also, remember that you can always e-mail me and ask for help. I will also be happy to get your feedback:

kira.novac@kiraglutenfreerecipes.com

Free Complimentary Recipe eBook

Before we jump into the recipes, I would love to offer you a free complimentary eBook that will give you even more gluten-free dessert ideas. While the book you are reading right now focuses <u>on vegan gluten-free recipes</u>, the one that I offer you as a special gift contains both vegan and paleo options.

Download your free recipe eBook here:

<u>http://bit.ly/gluten-free-desserts-book</u>

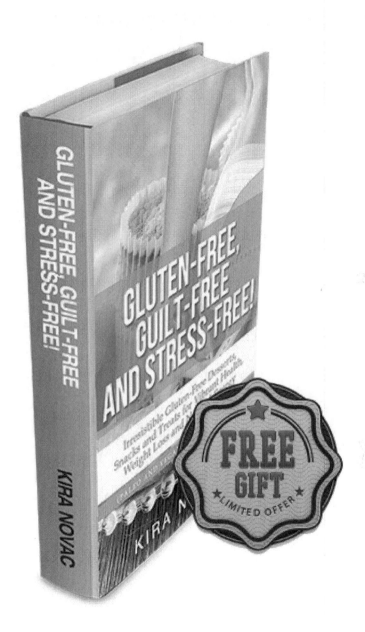

PART 1 Breakfast Recipes

Cinnamon Apple Overnight Oats

Servings: 4

Oats Ingredients:

- 2 cups of unsweetened almond milk
- 2 tablespoons of maple syrup
- 2 teaspoons of vanilla extract
- 2 cups of old-fashioned oats (gluten-free)
- 2 tablespoons of chia seeds
- 1 teaspoon of ground cinnamon
- Pinch of salt

Apple Topping Ingredients:

- 2 tablespoons of coconut oil
- 2 medium apples, cored and chopped
- 2 tablespoons of coconut sugar
- ½ teaspoon of ground cinnamon

- 1 ½ tablespoons of arrowroot powder

Instructions:

1. Whisk together your almond milk, maple syrup, and vanilla extract in a mixing bowl.
2. Add in the oats, chia seeds, cinnamon and the salt.
3. Whisk the ingredients together until they are combined fully.
4. Cover the bowl and chill the mixture in the fridge overnight.
5. In the morning, melt the coconut oil in a medium saucepan.
6. Add the apples, coconut sugar, and cinnamon.
7. Cook ingredients for 3 to 5 minutes on the medium heat setting until apples are tender.
8. Stir in your arrowroot powder and cook for another minute or so until thick.
9. Spoon the oats into bowls and top with the apple mixture to serve.

Spinach Green Apple Smoothie

Servings: 1

Ingredients:

- 2 cups of fresh chopped spinach
- 1 medium green apple, cored and diced
- 1 small stalk celery, sliced thin
- 1 cup of unsweetened apple juice
- ¼ cup of canned coconut milk
- 3 to 4 ice cubes
- 1 teaspoon of maple syrup

Instructions:

1. Combine your spinach and apple juice in a high-speed blender.
2. Pulse the mixture a few times then blend it until it is smooth.
3. Add in your celery, coconut milk, ice cubes and maple syrup.

4. Blend the smoothie ingredients until they are smooth and lump free.

5. Pour your smoothie into a glass and enjoy right away.

Coconut Flour Banana Pancakes

Servings: 6

Ingredients:

- ¼ cup of ground flaxseed
- ¾ cups of warm water
- ½ cup of sifted coconut flour
- 1 teaspoon of baking powder
- Pinch of salt
- 1 ¼ cups of unsweetened almond milk
- ½ tablespoon of vanilla extract
- 2 medium bananas, peeled and sliced

Instructions:

1. Whisk together your flaxseed and your water in a small bowl – let it rest for 5 minutes.
2. Combine your coconut flour, baking powder and salt in a mixing bowl.
3. Add in your almond milk and vanilla extract along with the flaxseed mixture.

4. Whisk your ingredients together until the batter is free from lumps – let rest 3 minutes.

5. Preheat a nonstick skillet over the medium heat setting.

6. Spoon your batter into the skillet using about ¼ cup of it for each pancake.

7. Add a few slices of banana into the wet batter and let it cook until the underside is browned.

8. Flip your pancakes and cook them for another minute or two until the underside browns.

9. Slide the finished pancakes onto a plate and repeat with the rest of the batter.

Almond Flour Raspberry Muffins

Servings: 12

Ingredients:

- 7 ounces of blanched almond flour
- 1/3 cup of ground flaxseed
- ½ teaspoon of baking soda
- ½ teaspoon of ground cinnamon
- Pinch of salt
- 10 ½ ounces of unsweetened applesauce
- ¼ cup of pure maple syrup
- 2 tablespoons of coconut oil, melted
- ½ teaspoon of vanilla extract
- 1 cup of fresh raspberries

Instructions:

1. Preheat your oven to a temperature of 350°F and line the cups of a muffin pan using paper liners.
2. Combine your almond flour and flaxseed in a mixing bowl with the baking soda, cinnamon and the salt.
3. In another bowl, stir together your applesauce and maple syrup with the coconut oil and the vanilla extract.

4. Stir your almond flour mixture into the applesauce mixture until all lumps are gone then fold in your raspberries.

5. Spoon your muffin batter into the muffin pan, filling each cup about ¾ full.

6. Bake your muffins until a knife you insert into the middle comes out clean – that will take about 28 to 32 minutes.

7. Cool your muffins in the pan for about 5 minutes then cool on wire racks.

Maple Blueberry Overnight Oats

Servings: 4

Ingredients:

- 2 cups of coconut milk
- 2 tablespoons of maple syrup
- 1 ½ teaspoons of vanilla extract
- 2 cups of old-fashioned oats (gluten-free)
- 1/3 cup slivered almonds
- 2 tablespoons of chia seeds
- Pinch of salt
- 1 to 2 cups of fresh blueberries

Instructions:

1. Whisk together your coconut milk, maple syrup, and vanilla extract in a mixing bowl.
2. Add in the oats, chia seeds, almonds and the salt.
3. Whisk the ingredients together until they are combined fully.

4. Cover the bowl and chill the mixture in the fridge overnight.

5. In the morning, spoon the oats into bowls and top with the blueberries to serve.

Tropical Mango Lime Smoothie

Servings: 1

Ingredients:

- 1 small frozen banana, peeled and sliced
- 1 cup of frozen chopped mango
- ½ cup of frozen pineapple chunks
- 1 fresh kiwi, peeled and sliced
- 1 cup of fresh squeezed orange juice
- ¼ cup of canned coconut milk
- 1 teaspoon of fresh lemon juice

Instructions:

1. Combine your banana, kiwi and orange juice in a high-speed blender.
2. Pulse the mixture a few times then blend it until it is smooth.
3. Add in your mango, pineapple, coconut milk, and lemon juice.

4. Blend the smoothie ingredients until they are smooth and lump free.

5. Pour your smoothie into a glass and enjoy right away.

Cranberry Orange Scones

Servings: 12

Ingredients:

- 3 cups of all-purpose gluten-free flour
- 1 tablespoon of baking powder
- ½ teaspoon of salt
- 2/3 cups of fresh squeezed orange juice
- ½ cup of pure maple syrup
- 1/3 cup of vegetable oil
- 2/3 cups of unsweetened dried cranberries
- ½ cup of chopped walnuts
- ¼ cup of fresh orange zest

Instructions:

1. Preheat your oven to a temperature of 425°F and line a cookie sheet with parchment.
2. Combine your gluten-free flour with your baking powder and salt in a mixing bowl.

3. In another bowl, whisk together your orange juice, maple syrup and vegetable oil.

4. Stir your orange juice mixture into your dry ingredients until the batter is free from lumps.

5. Fold in your cranberries and walnuts and stir in the orange zest.

6. Use a tablespoon to drop heaping spoonfuls of your scone batter onto your prepared cookie sheet.

7. Bake your scones for about 10 to 12 minutes until they are golden on the edges.

Spiced Pumpkin Almond Muffins

Servings: 12

Ingredients:

- 2 tablespoons of ground flaxseed
- 1/3 cup of warm water
- 2/3 cups of white rice flour
- ½ cup of buckwheat flour
- ½ cup of tapioca starch
- 1 teaspoon of pumpkin pie spice
- 1 teaspoon of baking soda
- ½ teaspoon of baking powder
- ½ teaspoon of salt
- 1 ¼ cups of pumpkin puree
- ¾ cups of pure maple syrup
- ½ cup of melted coconut oil
- ¼ cup of water, cold
- 1/3 cup finely chopped almonds

Instructions:

1. Preheat your oven to a temperature of 325°F and line the cups of a muffin pan using paper liners.

2. Whisk together your flaxseed and the water in a small bowl – let it rest for 5 minutes.

3. Combine your rice flour and buckwheat flour in a mixing bowl with the tapioca starch, pumpkin pie spice, baking soda, baking powder and salt.

4. In another bowl, stir together your pumpkin puree and maple syrup along with your coconut oil, water, and the flaxseed mixture.

5. Stir your dry ingredient mixture into the wet ingredient mixture until all lumps are gone then fold in your almonds.

6. Spoon your muffin batter into the muffin pan, filling each cup about ¾ full.

7. Bake your muffins until a knife you insert into the middle comes out clean – that will take about 40 to 45 minutes.

8. Cool your muffins in the pan for about 5 minutes then cool on wire racks.

Coconut Flour Cinnamon Waffles

Servings: 6

Ingredients:

- 2 tablespoons of ground flaxseed
- 1/3 cup of warm water
- 1 cup of gluten-free oat flour
- 5 tablespoons of coconut flour
- ½ cup of shredded unsweetened coconut
- 1 ½ teaspoons of baking powder
- ¾ teaspoons of ground cinnamon
- 1 ½ cups coconut milk
- ¼ cup of melted coconut oil
- 2 ½ tablespoons of pure maple syrup
- 1 teaspoon of vanilla extract

Instructions:

1. Preheat your waffle iron by following the manufacturer's instructions.

2. Whisk together your flaxseed and water in a small bowl then let it rest 5 minutes.

3. Combine your oat flour and coconut flour in a mixing bowl then stir in the coconut, baking powder and the cinnamon.

4. Stir in your coconut milk and coconut oil along with the maple syrup and vanilla extract.

5. Mix the ingredients until you have a smooth batter – it will be fairly thick.

6. Spoon the batter into your prepared waffle iron and cook it according to your manufacturer's instructions.

7. Remove the cooked waffle to a plate and repeat the process with the rest of your batter.

Blueberry Mint Smoothie

Servings: 1

Ingredients:

- 1 ½ cups of frozen or fresh blueberries
- 1 cup of fresh chopped spinach
- 1 cup of unsweetened almond milk
- ½ cup of ice cubes
- 2 tablespoons of fresh chopped mint
- 1 teaspoon of agave nectar

Instructions:

1. Combine your spinach and almond milk in a high-speed blender.
2. Pulse the mixture a few times then blend it until it is smooth.
3. Add in your blueberries, ice cubes, mint and agave.
4. Blend the smoothie ingredients until they are smooth and lump free.
5. Pour your smoothie into a glass and enjoy right away.

Cinnamon Blueberry Pancakes

Servings: 6

Ingredients:

- ¼ cup of ground flaxseed
- ¾ cups of warm water
- ½ cup of sifted coconut flour
- 1 teaspoon of baking powder
- Pinch of salt
- 1 ¼ cups of unsweetened almond milk
- ½ tablespoon of vanilla extract
- 1 cup of fresh blueberries

Instructions:

1. Whisk together your flaxseed and your water in a small bowl – let it rest for 5 minutes.
2. Combine your coconut flour, baking powder and salt in a mixing bowl.
3. Add in your almond milk and vanilla extract along with the flaxseed mixture.

4. Whisk your ingredients together until the batter is free from lumps – let rest 3 minutes.

5. Preheat a nonstick skillet over the medium heat setting.

6. Spoon your batter into the skillet using about ¼ cup of it for each pancake.

7. Add a few blueberries into the wet batter and let it cook until the underside is browned.

8. Flip your pancakes and cook them for another minute or two until the underside browns.

9. Slide the finished pancakes onto a plate and repeat with the rest of the batter.

Coconut Vanilla Muffins

Servings: 12

Ingredients:

- 7 ounces of blanched almond flour
- 1/3 cup of ground flaxseed
- ½ teaspoon of baking soda
- ½ teaspoon of ground cinnamon
- Pinch of salt
- 10 ½ ounces of unsweetened applesauce
- ¼ cup of pure maple syrup
- 2 tablespoons of coconut oil, melted
- 1 teaspoon of vanilla extract
- ½ cup of shredded unsweetened coconut

Instructions:

1. Preheat your oven to a temperature of 350°F and line the cups of a muffin pan using paper liners.
2. Combine your almond flour and flaxseed in a mixing bowl with the baking soda, cinnamon and the salt.

3. In another bowl, stir together your applesauce and maple syrup with the coconut oil, and your vanilla extract.

4. Stir your almond flour mixture into the applesauce mixture until all lumps are gone then fold in your shredded coconut.

5. Spoon your muffin batter into the muffin pan, filling each cup about ¾ full.

6. Bake your muffins until a knife you insert into the middle comes out clean -- that will take about 28 to 32 minutes.

7. Cool your muffins in the pan for about 5 minutes then cool on wire racks.

PART 2 Soup and Salad Recipes

Curried Butternut Squash Soup

Servings: 6

Ingredients:

- 1 (2-pound) butternut squash
- ½ tablespoon of olive oil
- 2 tablespoons of coconut oil
- 1 medium yellow onion, chopped
- 1 cup of chopped baby carrots
- 2 tablespoons of red curry paste
- 2 (14-ounce) cans of vegetable broth
- 2 small bay leaves
- ¼ cup of canned coconut milk

Instructions:

1. Preheat your oven to a temperature of 375°F.

2. Cut your squash in half and brush it with olive oil then put it in a glass baking dish.

3. Roast your squash for 1 hour until it is tender then cool it a little before scooping the flesh into a bowl.

4. Heat your coconut oil in a large saucepan on the medium-high heat setting.

5. Stir in your onions and carrots and cook for 4 to 5 minutes then stir in the curry paste.

6. Add your vegetable broth and three cups of the roasted squash.

7. Bring the mixture to a boil and then reduce the heat to medium-low.

8. Add the bay leaf and then simmer your soup for 1 hour.

9. Remove the saucepan from the heat and puree your soup using an immersion blender.

10. Whisk in your coconut milk and serve the soup hot.

Chopped Kale Salad

Servings: 4

Ingredients:

- 2 bunches of fresh kale, rinsed well
- ¼ cup of fresh squeezed lemon juice
- 3 ½ tablespoons of olive oil
- 2 teaspoons of minced garlic
- Salt and pepper to taste
- 1 cup of toasted pecan halves
- ½ small red onion, sliced thin

Instructions:

1. Trim the stems off the kale and chop it coarsely before placing it in a serving bowl.
2. Combine the lemon juice and olive oil with the garlic, salt and pepper in a food processor.
3. Blend the mixture well then toss it in with the chopped kale.

4. Top the kale salad with toasted pecans and sliced red onion to serve.

Cream of Broccoli Soup

Servings: 6

Ingredients:

- ¾ cups of raw cashew halves
- ½ tablespoon of coconut oil
- 2 medium yellow onions, chopped
- 2 large carrots, peeled and chopped
- 2 stalks celery, sliced
- Salt and pepper to taste
- 1 lbs. chopped broccoli florets
- 1 tablespoon of minced garlic
- 6 cups of water, divided

Instructions:

1. Soak your cashews in warm water for at least 30 minutes.
2. Heat your oil in a large saucepan on the medium-high heat setting.
3. Add in your onions and cook for 3 to 4 minutes.
4. Stir in your carrots and celery then season with salt and pepper to taste.

5. Cook the veggies for 5 minutes then stir in broccoli and garlic – cook 5 minutes more.

6. Stir in 5 cups of water and then bring the soup to a boil.

7. Reduce the heat to the low heat setting and simmer your soup for 15 minutes covered with a lid.

8. Drain the water from your cashews and then blend them with 1 cup of fresh water in a food processor until smooth.

9. Remove your soup from the heat and puree it using an immersion blender.

10. Whisk in your blended cashew mixture and then season the soup to taste.

Strawberry Balsamic Spinach Salad

Servings: 4

Ingredients:

- 6 cups of fresh chopped baby spinach
- 1 cup of sliced mushrooms
- ½ small red onion, sliced thin
- 1 ¼ cups of sliced strawberries (divided)
- 2 tablespoons of olive oil
- 1 tablespoon of balsamic vinegar
- Salt and pepper to taste

Instructions:

1. Toss together the spinach, mushrooms and red onion in a large salad bowl.
2. Combine your olive oil and balsamic vinegar in a food processor with ¼ cup of strawberries.
3. Blend the mixture smooth and then season with salt and pepper to taste.

4. Top the salad with the rest of the strawberries and drizzle with the dressing to serve.

Chilled Spicy Avocado Soup

Servings: 4

Ingredients:

- 1 large ripe avocado, pitted and chopped
- 1 ½ medium English cucumbers, peeled and diced
- 1 cup coconut yogurt
- 2 tablespoons of chopped chives
- 1 teaspoon of fresh lime juice
- 1 teaspoon of salt
- ½ small jalapeno, seeded and minced
- Pinch of cayenne pepper

Instructions:

1. Place your avocado in a food processor and blend it until it is smooth.
2. Add the rest of your ingredients and blend well.
3. Pour the soup into a serving bowl and chill it for at least an hour until cold.

4. Spoon the soup into bowls and sprinkle with paprika to serve.

Southwest-Style Corn and Bean Salad

Servings: 6

Ingredients:

- 2 (15-ounce) cans of black beans, rinsed and drained
- 1 (15-ounce) can of whole kernel corn, rinsed and drained
- 1 (14.5-ounce) can of diced tomatoes, rinsed and drained
- 1 small red onion, diced fine
- ¼ cup of fresh squeezed lime juice
- 2 tablespoons of olive oil
- 4 tablespoons of fresh chopped cilantro
- ½ jalapeno, seeded and minced
- Salt and pepper to taste
- 8 to 10 cups of fresh chopped lettuce

Instructions:

1. Combine your black beans, corn, tomato and red onion in a salad bowl.
2. In a separate bowl, whisk together your lime juice, olive oil, cilantro and jalapeno.

3. Season with salt and pepper to taste.

4. Toss the black bean mixture with the dressing and serve over chopped lettuce.

Thai Tofu and Vegetable Curry

Servings: 6

Ingredients:

- 2 ½ cups of vegetable broth (low sodium)
- 1 (14-ounce) can of coconut milk
- 1 ½ tablespoons of Thai red curry paste
- ¼ teaspoon ground ginger
- Salt to taste
- 10 ounces of sliced mushrooms
- ¼ lbs. of green beans, trimmed
- 1 cup of chopped carrots
- 1 medium sweet potato, peeled and chopped
- 1 (16-ounce) package extra-firm tofu, drained and chopped
- ¼ lbs. sugar snap peas
- 2 tablespoons of fresh lime juice
- 2 tablespoons of fresh chopped basil

Instructions:

1. Combine your vegetable broth, coconut milk and curry paste in a medium saucepan.
2. Whisk in your ginger and salt then bring the mixture to a boil.
3. Stir in your mushrooms, beans, carrots and sweet potato.
4. Simmer your vegetables for 5 minutes until they are just turning tender.
5. Stir in your tofu along with the snap peas and cook for 1 to 2 minutes more.
6. Add in your lime juice and basil then season with salt and pepper to taste.
7. Serve the curry hot over steamed rice, if desired.

Mango Mandarin Spinach Salad

Servings: 4

Ingredients:

- 6 cups of fresh chopped baby spinach, packed
- ¼ cup of extra-virgin olive oil
- 2 tablespoons of fresh lemon juice
- 1 teaspoon of agave nectar
- Salt and pepper to taste
- 1 cup of fresh chopped mango
- 1 cup of mandarin oranges, drained
- ¼ cup of toasted almonds

Instructions:

1. Place the spinach in a large salad bowl.
2. Whisk together your olive oil, lemon juice, agave, salt and pepper in a bowl.
3. Toss the spinach with the dressing and divide it among four salad plates.

4.   Top each salad with ¼ of the mango and mandarin oranges.

5.   Sprinkle the salads with toasted almonds to serve.

Chickpea and Cauliflower Stew

Servings: 6

Ingredients:

- 2 tablespoons of coconut oil
- 1 large yellow onion, chopped
- 2 teaspoons of ground cumin
- ¾ teaspoons of ground ginger
- Salt and pepper to taste
- 3 (14-ounce) cans diced tomatoes in juice
- 1 (15-ounce) can of chickpeas, rinsed and drained
- 1 ½ heads of cauliflower, chopped into florets
- ¾ cups of seedless raisins
- ¾ cups of water
- 4 cups of fresh chopped spinach

Instructions:

1. Heat your oil in a large saucepan on the medium heat setting.

2. Add in your onions and cook for 5 minutes until they start to soften.

3. Stir in your seasonings and cook for another minutes then add your tomatoes.

4. Add in your chickpeas and cauliflower along with the raisins.

5. Stir in the water and bring the stew mixture to a boil.

6. Reduce the heat and simmer the vegetables for 15 to 20 minutes until they are tender.

7. Stir in the spinach and cook for 1 minute more. Serve hot.

PART 3 Dinner Recipes

Mashed Sweet Potato Casserole

Servings: 8

Ingredients:

- 5 large sweet potatoes, peeled and chopped
- 1 cup old-fashioned oats (gluten-free)
- 1 ½ cups chopped almonds
- 1/3 cup of blanched almond flour
- 1 teaspoon of ground cinnamon
- ½ teaspoon of salt
- ¼ cup of melted coconut oil
- 2 tablespoons of maple syrup

Instructions:

1. Bring a large pot of salted water to boil and add your sweet potatoes.

2. Boil the sweet potatoes on the medium-high heat setting for 10 to 15 minutes until tender then drain well.

3. Preheat your oven to a temperature of 375°F and grease a 10-cup casserole dish.

4. Place your oats in a food processor and pulse to grind.

5. Transfer the oats to a bowl and stir in your almond flour, almonds, cinnamon and salt.

6. Stir in your coconut oil and maple syrup.

7. Mash your sweet potatoes with a potato masher along with the vegan butter then spread them in the baking dish.

8. Top the sweet potatoes with the oat mixture and bake for 15 to 22 minutes until heated through.

Skillet Fried BBQ Tofu

Servings: 6

Ingredients:

- 2 (14-ounce) packages extra-firm tofu
- 2 tablespoons coconut oil
- ½ cup vegan bbq sauce

Instructions:

1. Place the tofu on a plate and cover with a towel and a second plate – press the tofu for 30 minutes.
2. Preheat a large skillet on the medium-high heat setting while you slice the tofu.
3. Heat the oil in the skillet then add the tofu in a single layer.
4. Fry the tofu for 5 minutes or until browned then flip and fry for another 5 minutes.
5. Remove the skillet from the heat and toss in the BBQ sauce to serve.

Creamy Cauliflower Pasta Alfredo

Servings: 6

Ingredients:

- 6 cups of chopped cauliflower florets
- 1 tablespoon of olive oil
- 3 large cloves of garlic, minced
- ¾ cups of unsweetened almond milk
- 1/3 cup of nutritional yeast
- 1 ½ tablespoons of fresh lemon juice
- ½ teaspoon of onion powder
- ½ teaspoon of garlic powder
- Salt and pepper to taste
- 10 ounces of uncooked gluten-free pasta

Instructions:

1. Bring a large pot of salted water to a boil and then add in your cauliflower.
2. Boil the cauliflower for 4 to 6 minutes until it is tender then drain well.

3. Heat the oil in a large skillet on the low heat setting.

4. Add the garlic and cook for 5 minutes.

5. Transfer the garlic to a food processor and add the cauliflower.

6. Add the almond milk along with the nutritional yeast and lemon juice.

7. Blend in the onion powder, garlic powder, salt and pepper.

8. Bring another pot of salted water to boil and cook your pasta to al dente according to the directions on the package.

9. Drain the pasta and add it back to the pot – stir in the cauliflower sauce and cook until heated through.

Quinoa Veggie Burgers

Servings: 6

Ingredients:

- 1 tablespoon of ground flaxseed
- 3 tablespoons of warm water
- ¾ cups of cooked quinoa
- ½ cup fresh chopped spinach
- 5 tablespoons of oat flour (gluten-free)
- ¼ cup of shredded carrot
- 2 tablespoons of sundried tomatoes in oil, chopped
- 2 tablespoons of hulled sunflower seeds
- 2 tablespoons of fresh chopped basil
- 1 clove of minced garlic
- Salt and pepper to taste

Instructions:

1. Preheat your oven to a temperature of 400°F and line a cookie sheet with parchment.

2.   Whisk together your flaxseed and water in a small bowl –
     let rest for 5 minutes.

3.   Combine all of the remaining ingredients in a mixing bowl
     then stir in the flaxseed mixture.

4.   Shape the mixture into patties using about ¼ cup per
     patty.

5.   Place the patties on the cookie sheet and bake for 15
     minutes.

6.   Flip the patties and bake for another 10 minutes until
     browned. Serve hot.

Easy Shepherd's Pie with Gravy

Servings: 6

Ingredients:

- 3 lbs. of red potatoes, peeled and halved
- 1 tablespoon of olive oil
- 1 large yellow onion, chopped
- 1 tablespoon of minced garlic
- 1 ½ cups of diced carrots
- 1 cup of diced celery
- 1 cup of diced parsnips
- 2 tablespoons of vegan butter
- ½ cup of unsweetened almond milk
- Salt and pepper to taste
- 1 cup of vegetable broth
- ¼ cup of cooking sherry
- 3 tablespoons of gluten-free all-purpose flour

Instructions:

1. Preheat your oven to a temperature of 425°F and grease a casserole dish.
2. Place your potatoes in a pot of salted water and then bring it to a boil.
3. Simmer the potatoes on the low heat setting for 30 minutes until fork tender.
4. Heat the oil in a skillet on the medium heat setting.
5. Add the onion and garlic and cook for about 5 minutes until tender then stir in the remaining vegetables.
6. Cook the veggies for about 10 minutes until they are tender.
7. Drain the potatoes then place them back in the pot and mash them with the vegan butter and the almond milk.
8. Season the potatoes with salt and pepper to taste.
9. Whisk together your vegetable broth, sherry and gluten-free flour in a bowl.
10. Toss this mixture into the vegetables in the skillet and cook them for another 8 to 10 minutes.
11. Spread your vegetable mixture in the casserole dish and top with the mashed potatoes.
12. Bake for 35 minutes until hot and bubbling – cool 10 minutes before serving.

Grilled Tofu and Veggie Skewers

Servings: 6

Ingredients:

- 1 ½ tablespoons of rice vinegar
- 1 ½ tablespoons of tamari (gluten-free soy sauce)
- 1 tablespoon of sesame oil
- ¼ teaspoon of fresh ground pepper
- 1 (14-ounce) package extra-firm tofu, drained and cut into cubes
- 1 red bell pepper, cored and cut into 1-inch chunks
- 1 green bell pepper, cored and cut into 1-inch chunks
- 1 cup of cherry tomatoes
- 1 cup of button mushrooms
- 1 medium zucchini, cut into thick slices and halved
- Wooden skewers, soaked in water overnight

Instructions:

1. Whisk together your vinegar, tamari, sesame oil and pepper in a mixing bowl.

2. Toss in your tofu until coated then chill for 2 hours, tossing occasionally.

3. Preheat your grill to the high heat setting and brush the grates with oil.

4. Slide the tofu onto the skewers, alternating with the vegetables.

5. Place the skewers on the grill and cook for 5 minutes then turn the skewers.

6. Cook for another 5 minutes or until the tofu is cooked through and the veggies are slightly charred.

7. Serve the skewers hot with a side of steamed rice, if desired.

Spaghetti Squash with Sautéed Veggies

Servings: 4

Ingredients:

- 1 large spaghetti squash
- 1 tablespoon of olive oil
- 1 medium yellow onion, chopped
- 1 teaspoon of minced garlic
- 1 red bell pepper, cored and chopped
- 1 green bell pepper, cored and chopped
- 1 cup of diced zucchini
- ½ teaspoon of dried oregano
- Salt and pepper to taste

Instructions:

1. Preheat your oven to a temperature of 400°F.
2. Cut your squash in half and remove the seeds then place the squash halves cut-side down in a glass dish.
3. Pour in an inch of water then bake for 30 to 45 minutes until very tender.

4. Let the squash cool a little bit then shred the flesh into a bowl using a fork.

5. Heat the oil in a skillet on the medium-high heat setting.

6. Add the onion and garlic then cook for 6 to 8 minutes until tender.

7. Stir in the bell peppers and zucchini and cook for another 5 minutes.

8. Toss in the cooked spaghetti squash along with the oregano, salt and pepper.

9. Cook for 2 to 3 minutes until heated through and then serve.

Zucchini Pasta with Chunky Sauce

Servings: 4

Ingredients:

- 1 tablespoon of olive oil
- 1 large yellow onion, chopped
- 1 tablespoon of minced garlic
- Salt and pepper to taste
- 6 cups of diced tomatoes
- ½ cup of sundried tomatoes in oil
- 1 teaspoon of dried oregano
- 2 large zucchini, cut into noodle-like threads

Instructions:

1. Heat the oil in a medium skillet on the medium-high heat setting.
2. Stir in the onion and garlic then season with salt and pepper as you like.
3. Cook for 5 minutes until the onion is tender then stir in the tomatoes.

4. Bring the mixture to a boil on the medium-high heat setting then reduce to the medium setting and simmer for 15 minutes.

5. Place the sundried tomatoes in your food processor and add about 1 cup of the mixture from the skillet.

6. Blend smooth then stir the mixture back into the skillet and season with oregano, salt and pepper.

7. Heat another skillet over medium heat with a little bit of oil.

8. Add the zucchini noodles and cook until just heated through – serve hot with the sauce.

Vegan Enchilada Casserole

Servings: 8 to 10

Ingredients:

- ½ lbs. uncooked gluten-free noodles
- 1 tablespoon of olive oil
- 1 medium red onion, chopped
- 1 red bell pepper, cored and chopped
- 1 green bell pepper, cored and chopped
- 1 jalapeno, seeded and minced
- 3 tablespoons of taco seasoning
- 1 (15-ounce) can of black beans, rinsed and drained well
- 2 cups of enchilada sauce
- 6 green onions, sliced thin
- Salt and pepper to taste
- Salsa, to serve
- Chopped avocado, to serve

Instructions:

1. Preheat your oven to a temperature of 350°F and grease a glass baking dish.
2. Cook the pasta to al dente according to the direction then drain well.
3. Heat the oil in a large skillet on the medium-high heat setting.
4. Add the onions, peppers and jalapeno – sauté for about 8 minutes until tender.
5. Stir in the taco seasoning along with your beans and 1 cup of sauce.
6. Cook the mixture for 5 minutes then stir in your cooked pasta and green onion – season with salt and pepper as you like.
7. Spread about ½ cup of your enchilada sauce in the bottom of the baking dish and top with the mixture from the skillet.
8. Pour the remaining sauce over top and bake for 15 to 20 minutes until heated through.
9. Top the casserole with salsa and chopped avocado to serve.

Sweet Potato and Black Bean Burgers

Servings: 6

Ingredients:

- 1 large sweet potato, cut in half
- ½ cup canned blank beans, rinsed and drained
- ¾ cups of steamed brown rice
- ¼ cup of diced red onion
- ¼ cup of almond flour
- 1 teaspoon of ground cumin
- ¼ teaspoon of chili powder
- ¼ teaspoon of salt

Instructions:

1. Preheat your oven to a temperature of 400°F and place your sweet potatoes on a baking sheet lined with foil.
2. Bake your sweet potatoes for 30 minutes then reduce the oven temperature to 375°F.
3. Place your beans in a mixing bowl and mash them slightly with a fork.

4. Scoop the sweet potato out of the skins and stir it into the mashed bean mixture along with the rice, onion and almond flour.

5. Stir in your cumin, chili powder, salt and pepper until well combined.

6. Spoon the mixture onto a parchment-lined baking sheet, using about ¼ cup per scoop.

7. Flatten the scoops and bake the burgers for about 35 to 45 minutes, flipping once halfway through the cooking.

8. Serve the burgers hot on toasted vegan hamburger buns.

Lemon Dill Fried Tofu Slices

Servings: 4

Ingredients:

- 1/3 cup fresh lemon juice
- 2 tablespoons of tahini
- 2 tablespoons of water
- 1 cup fresh chopped dill
- 2 cloves minced garlic
- 2 (14-ounce) packages of extra-firm tofu, drained
- 2 tablespoons of coconut oil

Instructions:

1. Combine the lemon juice, tahini, and water in a food processor.
2. Add the fresh dill and garlic then blend until smooth and well combined.
3. Place the tofu on a plate and cover with a towel and a second plate – press the tofu for 30 minutes.

4. Preheat a large skillet on the medium-high heat setting while you slice the tofu.

5. Heat the oil in the skillet then add the tofu in a single layer.

6. Fry the tofu for 5 minutes or until browned then flip and fry for another 5 minutes.

7. Remove the skillet from the heat and toss in the lemon dill sauce to serve.

PART 4 Side Dish Recipes

Garlic Sautéed Broccoli Florets

Servings: 6

Ingredients:

- 3 tablespoons of olive oil
- 1 tablespoon of minced garlic
- 6 cups of chopped broccoli florets
- Salt and pepper to taste

Instructions:

1. Heat the oil in a large skillet on the medium-low heat setting.
2. Add your garlic and cook it for 1 minute until it is fragrant.
3. Toss in your broccoli florets and season with salt and pepper as needed.
4. Sauté the broccoli for 5 to 6 minutes until it turns bright green. Serve hot.

Chile-Lime Snow Peas

Servings: 6

Ingredients:

- 1 ½ lbs. of snow peas, trimmed
- Salt and pepper to taste
- 1 ½ tablespoons of olive oil
- 6 tablespoons of fresh chopped cilantro
- 6 tablespoons of roasted almonds, chopped
- 1 jalapeno, seeded and minced
- 1 teaspoon fresh lime zest

Instructions:

1. Fill a large saucepan with water and bring it to boil – add a little salt.
2. Add your snow peas to the pot of boiling water and cook for 1 to 2 minutes until they are just tender.
3. Immediately transfer the peas to a bowl of ice water to stop the cooking.
4. Drain the snow peas and pat them dry with paper towels.

5. Place the snow peas in a serving bowl and toss them with the olive oil, cilantro, almonds, jalapeno, and lime zest.

6. Serve the salad immediately.

Southern-Style Collard Greens

Servings: 6 to 8

Ingredients:

- 6 slices vegan bacon
- 1 tablespoon olive oil
- 1 medium Vidalia onion, chopped
- 1 tablespoon minced garlic
- 6 cups of vegetable broth
- 1 ½ lbs. of fresh collard greens, rinsed and trimmed
- 3 tablespoons of cider vinegar
- 2 teaspoons of coconut sugar
- Salt and pepper to taste

Instructions:

1. Cook the bacon in a skillet over medium heat until it is crisp then chop it up.
2. Heat the oil in a deep skillet on the medium heat setting.
3. Add in the onion and cook for 6 to 7 minutes until it is tender.

4. Stir in your garlic and cook for 1 minute.

5. Add your vegetable broth along with the collard greens, vinegar, and sugar – season the mixture with salt and pepper to taste.

6. Reduce the heat to low and cook for 2 hours until the collards are tender.

7. Serve the collard greens hot topped with chopped bacon.

Maple-Glazed Baby Carrots

Servings: 6 to 8

Ingredients:

- 2 tablespoons of coconut oil
- 2 ¼ cups of water
- 1 ½ tablespoons of sugar
- 1 teaspoon of salt
- 2 lbs. of baby carrots
- 3 tablespoons of vegan butter
- ¼ cup of pure maple syrup

Instructions:

1. Melt the coconut oil in a large saucepan over the medium heat setting.
2. Whisk in the water, sugar and salt then stir in the baby carrots.
3. Cover the saucepan and bring the mixture to a boil in the medium-high heat setting.

4. Reduce the heat setting to medium-low and simmer it for 10 minutes then drain well.

5. Melt the vegan butter in a large skillet on the medium-high heat setting.

6. Stir in your maple syrup until it is melted.

7. Toss in your carrots and cook for 5 minutes until they are hot.

Rosemary Roasted Veggie Medley

Servings: 6 to 8

Ingredients:

- 2 large sweet potatoes, peeled and chopped
- 2 large carrots, peeled and chopped
- 2 medium yellow onions, cut into quarters
- 1 medium parsnip, peeled and chopped
- 1 medium zucchini, cut into large chunks
- 1 head broccoli, cut into florets
- 1 head cauliflower, cut into florets
- 3 tablespoons olive oil
- 1 tablespoon dried rosemary
- ¼ cup of vegetable broth
- Salt and pepper to taste

Instructions:

1. Preheat your oven to a temperature of 350°F.
2. Toss together all of your vegetables in a large mixing bowl with the olive oil and rosemary.

3. Spread the vegetable mixture in a large glass baking dish and season with salt and pepper to taste.

4. Drizzle the vegetables with vegetable broth, tossing to coat.

5. Roast the vegetables for 15 minutes then stir them with a spatula or large spoon.

6. Let the veggies roast for another 15 to 20 minutes until they are tender.

Carrot Red Onion Slaw

Servings: 6

Ingredients:

- 2 lbs. carrots cut into matchsticks
- ½ small red onion, sliced thin
- ½ cup of fresh chopped cilantro
- 2 ½ tablespoons of olive oil
- 1 ½ tablespoons of lemon juice
- 2 teaspoons apple cider vinegar
- 1 teaspoon of maple syrup
- Salt and pepper to taste

Instructions:

1. Bring a large pot of salted water to a boil then add the carrots.
2. Cook the carrots for 1 to 2 minutes until tender then transfer to an ice water bath.
3. Drain the carrots well and transfer them to a bowl – add in the red onions and cilantro.

4. Whisk together the rest of your ingredients in a small bowl.

5. Toss your carrot and red onion mixture with the dressing and chill until you are ready to serve it.

PART 5 Snack and Dessert Recipes

Avocado Chocolate Mousse

Servings: 6

Ingredients:

- 3 medium avocadoes, pitted and chopped
- 3 tablespoons of unsweetened almond milk
- ½ cup of unsweetened cocoa powder
- 1 teaspoon of chia seeds
- ½ cup of agave nectar
- 1 teaspoon of vanilla extract

Instructions:

1. Place your chopped avocados in a food processor.
2. Add your almond milk and cocoa powder along with the chia seeds, agave and vanilla extract.
3. Blend the mixture until it is smooth and fully combined.
4. Spoon the mousse into dessert cups and chill at least 30 minutes before you serve it.

Sesame Kale Chips

Servings: 4

Ingredients:

- 2 bunches of fresh kale, stems trimmed and chopped
- 3 to 4 tablespoons of olive oil
- 2 tablespoons of fresh lemon juice
- 1/3 cup of sesame seeds
- Salt to taste

Instructions:

1. Preheat your oven to a temperature of 200°F.
2. Toss your chopped kale with the olive oil and lemon juice.
3. Spread the kale on parchment-lined baking sheets and sprinkle it with sesame seeds and salt.
4. Bake for 30 minutes then carefully flip the kale and bake another 20 minutes.
5. Cool the chips completely and then store in an airtight container.

Lemon Lime Sorbet

Servings: 6 to 8

Ingredients:

- 2 cups of water
- 2 cups of superfine sugar
- 1 cup of fresh lemon juice
- 1 cup of fresh lime juice
- 1 tablespoon of fresh lemon zest
- 2 teaspoons of fresh lime zest

Instructions:

1. Whisk together your water and sugar in a saucepan on the medium heat setting.
2. Once the sugar has dissolved, stir it in then remove the pot from the heat.
3. Cool the mixture to room temperature then whisk in your lemon juice, lime juice, lemon zest and lime zest.
4. Pour the mixture into your ice cream maker and freeze it according to the manufacturer's instructions.

5.   Once the sorbet is frozen, transfer it to a plastic container and freeze until ready to serve.

Dairy-Free Artichoke Dip

Servings: 6 to 8

Ingredients:

- 1 (14-ounce) can of artichoke hearts, drained
- 1 cup of canned white cannellini beans, drained well
- 4 tablespoons of nutritional yeast
- 3 tablespoons of water
- 2 tablespoons of cider vinegar
- 1 ½ tablespoons of olive oil
- 1 teaspoon of minced garlic
- 1 ½ cups of frozen spinach, thawed and squeezed to remove water
- Salt and pepper to taste

Instructions:

1. Place half of your artichokes in a food processor along with the beans, nutritional yeast, water and vinegar.
2. Blend the mixture until it is smooth and creamy.

3. Heat the oil in a skillet on the medium heat setting and add the garlic – cook 1 minute.

4. Stir in your spinach and cook for 1 minute.

5. Transfer the mixture in the food processor into a bowl and stir in the spinach and garlic mixture.

6. Chop the remaining artichokes and stir them in then season with salt and pepper to taste.

Almond Apple Crisp

Servings: 6

Ingredients:

- 6 medium ripe apples, peeled and sliced thin
- 6 tablespoons of maple syrup, divided
- 1 tablespoon of lemon juice
- 1 ½ teaspoons of ground cinnamon, divided
- ½ cup of blanched almond flour
- ½ cup of old-fashioned oats (gluten-free)
- ¼ cup of chopped almonds
- ¼ teaspoon of salt
- 3 tablespoons of vegan butter

Instructions:

1. Preheat your oven to 375°F and grease a pie plate with oil.
2. Combine your apples in a mixing bowl with 2 tablespoons maple syrup, lemon juice and 1 teaspoon ground cinnamon.
3. Spread your apples in the pie plate and set aside.

4. In another bowl, combine your almond flour and oats with the almonds, ½ teaspoon cinnamon and the salt.

5. Cut in your vegan butter and the remaining maple syrup until it forms a crumbled mixture.

6. Spread the mixture over your apples in the pie plate and bake for 30 to 35 minutes until browned.

7. Cool for at least 10 minutes before you serve the crisp.

Chocolate Chia Seed Pudding

Servings: 6

Ingredients:

- 2 ¼ cups of unsweetened almond milk
- ½ cup of chia seeds
- 1/3 cup of unsweetened cocoa powder
- ¼ cup of maple syrup
- 1 teaspoon of vanilla extract
- Pinch of salt

Instructions:

1. Combine the almond milk and chia seeds in a food processor.
2. Blend the mixture well then add in the cocoa powder, maple syrup, vanilla extract and salt.
3. Blend again until the mixture is well combined then pour into a bowl.
4. Cover and chill the pudding overnight then spoon into bowls to serve.

No-Bake Coconut Date Balls

Servings: 12

Ingredients:

- 1 cup of raw cashew halves
- ½ cup of shredded unsweetened coconut
- 1 cup of pitted Medjool dates
- 1 tablespoon of coconut oil
- ½ teaspoon of vanilla extract
- Pinch of salt

Instructions:

1. Combine the cashews and coconut in a food processor and blend until crumbled.
2. Add in your dates and coconut oil along with the vanilla extract and salt.
3. Blend the mixture until it is sticky and sticks together.
4. Shape the mixture into 12 round balls by hand and chill until firm.
5. Roll the balls in cocoa powder, if desired, before serving.

Cherry Lime Granita

Servings: 6 to 8

Ingredients:

- 2 ½ cups of fresh pitted cherries
- 1 cup of water
- 1 cup of superfine sugar
- 4 large limes, juiced

Instructions:

1. Place the cherries in a food processor and blend to puree.
2. Strain the cherry mixture through a mesh sieve, collecting the juice.
3. Whisk together your water and sugar in a small saucepan on the medium-high heat setting.
4. Bring the mixture to boil then stir well until the sugar is dissolved.
5. Remove your saucepan from the heat and whisk in your cherry juice and lime juice.
6. Chill the mixture overnight then pour in a large glass baking dish.

7.   Freeze the dish for 1 hour then stir gentle.

8.   Repeat the process, freezing and stirring every hour until the granite is frozen.

Cinnamon Baked Apple Chips

Servings: 6

Ingredients:

- 5 large ripe apples, cored and sliced thin
- Ground cinnamon, as needed

Instructions:

1. Preheat your oven to a temperature of 220°F and line cookie sheets with parchment.
2. Spread your apples on the cookie sheets in a single layer and sprinkle with cinnamon.
3. Bake the apple slices for 1 hour then flip and bake for another hour.
4. Turn off the oven and let the chips cool completely then store in an airtight container.

Cinnamon Blueberry Crumble

Servings: 6

Ingredients:

- 5 cups of fresh blueberries
- 6 tablespoons of maple syrup, divided
- 1 tablespoon of lemon juice
- 1 ½ teaspoons of ground cinnamon, divided
- ½ cup of blanched almond flour
- ½ cup of old-fashioned oats (gluten-free)
- ¼ cup of chopped pecans
- ¼ teaspoon of salt
- 3 tablespoons of vegan butter

Instructions:

1. Preheat your oven to 375°F and grease a pie plate with oil.
2. Combine your blueberries in a mixing bowl with 2 tablespoons maple syrup, lemon juice and 1 teaspoon ground cinnamon.
3. Spread your blueberries in the pie plate and set aside.

4. In another bowl, combine your almond flour and oats with the pecans, ½ teaspoon cinnamon and the salt.

5. Cut in your vegan butter and the remaining maple syrup until it forms a crumbled mixture.

6. Spread the mixture over your blueberries in the pie plate and bake for 30 to 35 minutes until browned.

7. Cool for at least 10 minutes before you serve the crisp.

Spicy Guacamole Dip

Servings: 6

Ingredients:

- 4 ripe avocadoes, pitted and chopped
- 1 medium red onion, diced fine
- 1 jalapeno, seeded and minced
- 1 tablespoon of minced garlic
- 1 bunch of fresh chopped cilantro
- ¾ teaspoons of ground cumin
- Salt and pepper to taste
- ¼ cup of fresh lime juice

Instructions:

1. Place the avocados in a mixing bowl and mash them with a fork.
2. Stir in your onion and jalapeno along with the tomatoes.
3. Add your garlic and cilantro, stirring the mixture until well combined.

4. Season your guacamole with the cumin, salt and pepper then stir in the lime juice.

5. Serve the guacamole dip immediately.

Sweet Citrus Sorbet

Servings: 6 to 8

Ingredients:

- 2 cups of water
- 2 cups of superfine sugar
- 1 cup of fresh orange juice
- ½ cup of fresh grapefruit juice
- ½ cup of fresh lemon juice
- 1 tablespoon of fresh lemon zest

Instructions:

1. Whisk together your water and sugar in a saucepan on the medium heat setting.
2. Once the sugar has dissolved, stir it in then remove the pot from the heat.
3. Cool the mixture to room temperature then whisk in your orange juice, grapefruit juice, lemon juice, and lemon zest.
4. Pour the mixture into your ice cream maker and freeze it according to the manufacturer's instructions.

5. Once the sorbet is frozen, transfer it to a plastic container and freeze until ready to serve.

Before you go, I'd like to remind you that there is a free, complimentary eBook waiting for you. Download it today to treat yourself to healthy, <u>gluten-free desserts and snacks</u> so that you never feel deprived again!

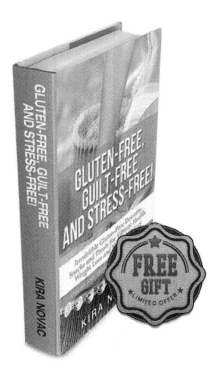

Download link

<u>http://bit.ly/gluten-free-desserts-book</u>

Conclusion

While the gluten-free diet is a medical treatment for individuals with celiac disease or gluten intolerance, it can be beneficial for nearly everyone. Before you decide whether the gluten-free diet is the right choice for you, take the time to learn as much as you can about the diet including its benefits, its risks, and which foods you can and cannot eat. Check out my website for more information where you will find the food lists and recipes to get started:

http://www.kiraglutenfreerecipes.com

There are different kinds of gluten-free diets (for example Paleo, vegetarian, vegan). You don't have to go 100% vegan to enjoy a gluten-free diet as it can be personalized. It's totally up to you. However, I believe that we should all learn more vegan options and reduce the consumption of animal products. This does not have to be painful as there are many delicious, plant-based options out there.

My main focus, as an author, is to create helpful and information gluten-free and anti-inflammatory recipe books that can accommodate vegans, vegetarians and paleo diet enthusiasts. I am always open to new suggestions so if you are looking for anything specific, please send me an e-mail and let me know.

I am here to help!

kira.novac@kiraglutenfreerecipes.com

One more thing- Me and my family follow gluten-free diets (a few years ago my son was diagnosed with celiac, also called celiac sprue, disease and, so we had to go gluten-free), and we also have close family members and friends who are vegan. This is why I had to learn how to combine both diets so that we can enjoy healthy and delicious meals together. Thanks to my vegan friends, I also realized that I need to reduce the consumption of animal products and discover more vegan options.

If you decide that the gluten-free diet is the diet for you and you also want to keep it vegan, I hope you will try some of the recipes in this book as you transition into the diet. Please let me know your favorites- the review section of this book is an excellent place to share your experience with other readers.

To post an honest review, please check <u>the review section of this book</u> is an excellent place to share your experience with other readers.

To post an honest review

One more thing... If you have received any value from this book, can you please rank it and post a short review? It only takes a few seconds really and it would really make my day. It's you I am writing for and your opinion is always much appreciated. In order to do so;

1. Log into your account
2. Search for my book on Amazon or check your orders/ or go to my author page at:

http://amazon.com/author/kira-novac

3. Click on a book you have read, then click on "reviews" and "create your review".

Please let me know your favorite motivational tip you learned from this book.

I would love to hear from you!

Recommended Reading

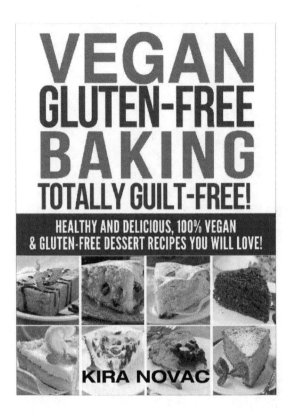

Book Link:

http://bit.ly/vegan-gf-baking

Recommended Reading

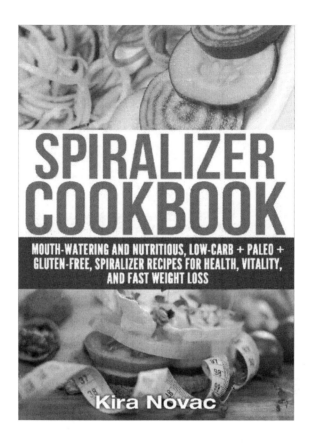

Book Link:

http://bit.ly/spiralizer-book

FOR MORE HEALTH BOOKS (KINDLE & PAPERBACK) BY KIRA NOVAC PLEASE VISIT:

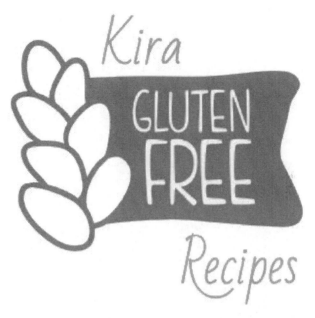

www.kiraglutenfreerecipes.com/books

Thank you for taking an interest in my work,

Kira and Holistic Wellness Books

HOLISTIC WELLNESS & HEALTH BOOKS

If you are interested in health, wellness, spirituality and personal development, visit our page and be the first one to know about free and 0.99 eBooks:

www.HolisticWellnessBooks.com

Made in the USA
San Bernardino, CA
10 May 2018